How To Swim
in Cold Water

How To Swim in Cold Water

(Natural vitality)

Børge B. N. Blåtind

Rev. date: 11/05/2013

To order additional copies of this book, contact:
Xlibris LLC
1-888-795-4274
www.Xlibris.com
Orders@Xlibris.com
142822

Contents

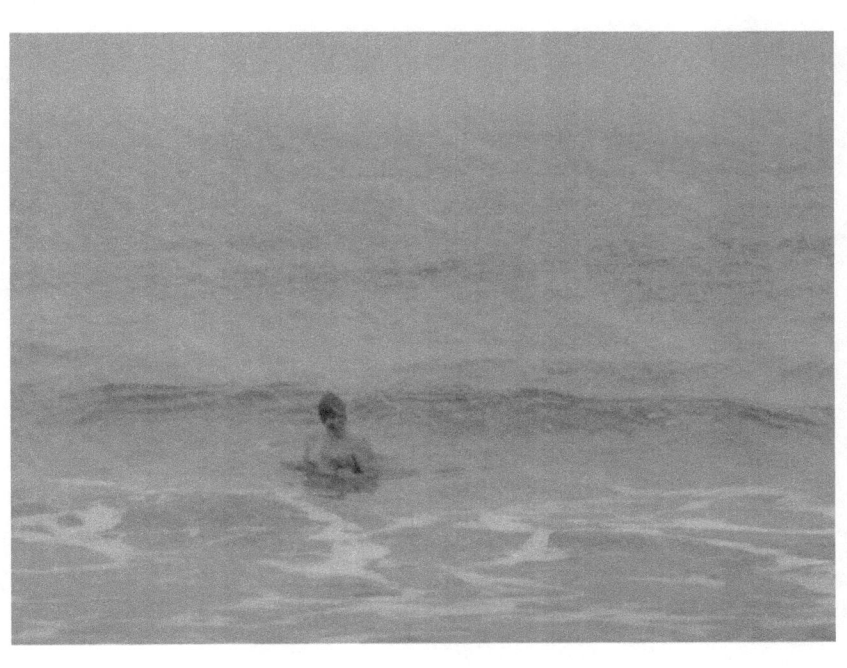

Thanks:
To my lovely wife Ezza and my two princesses Bella and Brenda
for their love and support and coming to the beach with me.

Also thanks to the professional and caring people at Xlibris for
publishing my books.

1. WORD OF CAUTION

IN THIS BOOK I have intentionally tried to be brief and to the point, so you can get a quick and functional introduction to the practices this book is about. By reading this manual you can safely proceed and have the trust you need for engaging in this experience. This is not a book you read for enjoyment, this is a manual. The goal for a manual is to teach you a skill or the way of doing something. This manual can teach you how be more relaxed in experiencing the pain of going into cold water, make you more relaxed and open to creative thoughts, becoming a man (or woman) of interest.

You may have read many "self help books" before, you understand what the authors say and feel that they are talking to you. You might wonder why those around you do not understand your talk and you attend new seminars where you nod and smile. You may thought you were going to take permanently lodging in these mindset, you were there, you experienced the "truth". Sadly you can not claim it by listening or reading any truth. Truth that lead to wisdom can be understood but to permanently claim it, is hard.

This book is NOT like this. This is a book of doing. Going into the icy cold water for the first time, really stop time, there is no faking, YOU are confronted with YOU.

Read the book, do the cold water first, then practicing it for a while, then do the Valø stones. The experiences you have is yours, big or small, they are yours.

. . . .

WARNING

No book like this can be without a warning. Here it comes;

Do not start any of these exercises without being allowed by your doctor, your psychologist, your psychiatrist, spouse, father, mother and friends. I say this a bit jokingly, as a friendly warning, but for you to take responsibility for your own development.

To work with the mind and body is fraught with danger, as a plethora of other pursuits we do, life is dangerous. If you have a mental illness, then I'm not sure if you have the ability right now to vitalize yourself. You can read the whole book and evaluate it yourself. Again, ask professionals for advice.

That being said, not all professionals or for that matter anyone are able to walk life's path for you. You have to walk it yourself.

The alternative is yes – you can. It is a dangerous thought.

2. INTRODUCTION

YOU MAY HAVE seen on TV people in arctic countries wade or jump into icy waters. You look at it and compare it to when you went for a relaxed swim in a heated pool, in a warm lake or sea, and comparing this to what you now see on TV seem like madness.

So first I must explain that the two situations you compare are NOT comparable. It is really not in any way the same, except in both you get wet. Going into cold water have nothing to do with what you generally talk about as "going for a swim".

Also there are various ways to do it, here are the three most common:

1. You travel to the beach, undress and wade slowly into the sea to chest level, and dip down to neck and stay like this as long as you can, maybe 20 seconds, then you stand up and still have water to chest level and repeat 4-7 times before slowly walking ashore and dress.
2. You travel to the sea or lake, undress and jump into the sea. Then you swim, usually 20 strokes and climb ashore and dress.
3. You have access to a sauna and sit in it until you are really heated up and then run down to the water and jump or wade into it. Then you swim, usually 20 strokes, climb ashore and run up and into the sauna. This is done once or repeated many times, sometimes for an hour or more.

I do the number one, and this handbook is about that experience. But I will briefly discuss the other two.

There is a danger in **jumping** into cold water, because when you jump and go totally under the body's circulation MAY switch from the larger to the smaller circulation and as blood is not fed to the brain you faint. Then you die.

WARNING!

So my advice is DO NOT JUMP into cold water. Even in summer people die here as they are out in a boat, maybe have drunk a beer, want to pee and slip and fall into the water. The body may then switch to the small circulation system and they faint and drown.

Wikipedia.org

The actual cause of death in cold water are usually the lethal *bodily reactions* to heat loss and to freezing water, rather than hypothermia (loss of core temperature). For example, plunged into freezing seas, around 20% of victims die within 2 minutes from *cold shock* (uncontrolled *rapid breathing* and gasping causing water inhalation, massive increase in blood pressure and cardiac strain leading to *cardiac arrest*, and *panic*), another 50% die within 15-30 minutes from *cold incapacitation* (inability to use or control limbs and hands for swimming or gripping, as the body 'protectively' shuts down the peripheral muscles of the limbs to protect its core), and exhaustion and unconsciousness cause *drowning*, claiming the rest within a similar time.

So my advice is **not** to do number 2, and if engaging in number 3 only wade into the water, never jump. Doing number 3 can have a stronger endorphin rush than number 1, still doing it in my prescribed way I have not experienced any bad things and even doing it having a cold have not aggravated the condition (probably not advisable to do it being sick).

I have done number 3 several times, but mostly going from the sauna into the snow outside and "swim" in the snow and rub yourself with the snow. I have also been once where we waded into water, but the experience is NOT the same as number 1 (witch this book is about). It gives you a burning sensation on the skin and when repeated many times you release a lot of endorphins and it gives you a really nice experience. It is like you see the world in colour for the first time.

Wikipedia.org

> Endorphins ("endogenous *morphine*") are *endogenous opioid peptides* that function as *neurotransmitters.* They are produced by the *pituitary gland* and the *hypothalamus* in *vertebrates* during *exercise,* excitement, *pain, consumption of spicy food, love* and *orgasm,* and they resemble the *opiates* in their abilities to produce *analgesia* and a feeling of well-being.

For this to happen it has to be repeated many times, hot 5-10 min, cold 3-4 min and so on and on. This as all should be done together with a friend and remember to drink lukewarm fresh water to compensate for your sweating.

. . . .

Now I have explained the physical act of going into the icy cold water, the different ways people do it, and the danger if doing it the wrong way.

But my friend, do not stop reading now, do not let your fear and imagination stop you from reading the whole book. There are so much more to it and why would people repeatedly do it 1-3 times a week all winter long? There must be a REASON?

Well, continue reading.

3. PREPARATION

WHY WOULD ANYBODY expose themselves to this cold water? Many do it one to three times a week all winter from September to May, what is the possible benefit? Or dare I say fun?

Below are some writings cut from wikipedia.org:

Wikipedia.org

> **Cryotherapy** is the local or general use of low temperatures in medical therapy. Cryotherapy is used to treat a variety of benign and malignant *lesions*. The term "cryotherapy" comes from the Greek *cryo* (κρύο) meaning *cold*, and *therapy* (θεραπεία) meaning *cure*. Cryotherapy has been used as early as the seventeenth century. Its goal is to decrease

cellular metabolism, increase cellular survival, decrease *inflammation*, decrease *pain* and spasm, promote *vasoconstriction*, and when using extreme temperatures, to destroy cells by crystallizing the *cytosol*. The most prominent use of the term refers to the surgical treatment, specifically known as *cryosurgery*. Other therapies that use the term are cryogenic chamber therapy and ice pack therapy.

Patients report that the experience is invigorating and improves a variety of conditions such as psychological stress, insomnia, *rheumatism*, muscle and joint pain, *fibromyalgia*, *itching*, and *psoriasis*. The immediate effect of skin cooling and analgesia lasts for 5 minutes, but the release of endorphins can have a lasting effect, where the pains and signs of inflammation as found in blood tests remain suppressed for weeks. The effects of extreme cold and endorphin release are scientifically studied.

However if ice pack therapy is applied for less than 10 minutes, performance can occur without detrimental effects. The physiological effects that the body goes through after cold therapy application include initial *vasoconstriction*, shunting all blood away from the body part, followed by *vasodilation*, as blood flows back to the affected area in attempt to re-warm. If the ice bag therapy is removed at this time, sportsmen are sent back to training or competition directly with no decrease in performance. Therefore, ice pack therapy is beneficial for injured athletes. as well as healthy athletes.

I am sure that if this aspect interest you specifically, there are much to be read. There are more to it than the health benefit as my book will show you, but these clippings above show that there have been done much research into cold treatment.

Here is what you need for your first go:

1. First find a place to do it, a clean beach, a clean lake or a clean river, preferable a beautiful spot.
2. The best is sea because of the properties of salt water and it is generally clean. It is good for the skin and have waves that break on you.
3. Have clothes that you can put on fast, the best is wool direct on body and woolen socks is a must. Do not wear cotton as it have no insulation when moist.
4. Outside of the wool can be anything (like a lined coverall), depend what you are doing afterwards.
5. Boots must be big so feet in woolen socks are not cramped.

6. Woolen hat that you also may wear going into water.
7. Get a big towel, women usually sew it as a tube so you can undress without exposing yourself.
8. Swimsuit to your liking.
9. Plastic sandals so you don't cut feet since when they are cold you don't feel when treading on shells and such.
10. A big nylon bag to keep clothes when you are undressed, so clothes don't get wet by snow, hail or rain, or are blown away.
11. A small rubber mat to stand on while changing.
12. Waterproof flashlight, and maybe a thermometer (most like to keep a log of the water-temperature the first year for fun, but as years go, most don't care).
13. Make sure your friend that come along is no idiot or prankster, as it is not funny if he hide your cloth or in any way is an asshole. It can even be dangerous, better alone then.

Do make an effort in finding a beautiful spot and for those of you living in more dangerous areas it must be safe. So most important is to do it where it is safe, and when it is safe. This is to become a fantastic weekly experience for you, so do find THE spot and find at least one person to join you.

First, you have nothing to fear from the experience, you don't have to be particularly fit and most that start to do it are women over the age of 40. I have met women and men between age of 40 and 85, I started at 36 and are now (2013) 57 years young. I have taken probably around 35 people over the years along, most do it once or a few times and maybe half have continued doing it. There have never been any ill effect on them, even people coming from tropical countries and just wanted a viking experience.

I like personally best to do it after dark, for various reasons; it get dark early here in winter time, it is also very quiet where I go and I get to see the air (I will write about that later). Another very beautiful thing you can experience (seldom) at nights in early winter is marine phosphorescence. It is an algae giving out light when touched (remember the film "PI"). So standing up in the water and seeing liquid light flow off your body is just beautiful. First time I am sure even the hardened among us will cry.

But going on a sunday morning, with lazy waves breaking and wading into the water is also just beautiful.

So you know a little of the proposed health benefit (scientifically), you have got the gear and found a spot. Now I have to speak a little of Pain and Fear.

Yes, there is pain as most of you have never experienced, when first wading to your knees and the water is between 4 and 7 deg Celsius there is pain. It is a bone-crushing pain and with that comes fear. You just want to run out of the water, put on the clothes and say (maybe scream) "this is madness/ too much/ I will NEVER do it/ I can not do it". The fear is just tangible, like a scream in your head. Actually it is difficult to differentiate between the pain and the fear.

My own saying; You can if you do it.

So if you do this with a friend that has also never done it, you have to encourage each other, walk in a little at a time, but not walk 1 m in and then run back to beach (again and again). Walk and breath, do not talk, do deep abdominal breathing, concentrate only on walking slowly and safely into the water (where you know there are no holes or hidden dangers). The pain will slowly (if you relax and let it) stop all internal dialogue (also called thinking) and maybe for the first time in your life you are HERE – Present.

When water reach your pubic areas a new pain come, but continue to walk so water reach between your nipples and bellybutton (solar plexus). Stay there at least 15-25 seconds (time goes REALLY slow now), look around, let the whole situation sink in and bend knees so water reach chin (if you want to take head under it is best to use earplugs as it is easy to get ear infection, and of-cause then no hat). First time just fill lungs and belly with air (try to be as big as you can, belly out) and hold breath and lower yourself to chin and stay at least 20 seconds before standing up with water to solar plexus. Repeat 3 times.

Then you slowly walk back to shore. Rub yourself a little with the towel and dress slowly.

While dressing you should feel no cold, it can be snowing and you are there just in your swimming suit feeling no cold, no pain. Do not be deceived, dress calmly and purposefully for 5 min after going out of water you may start freezing, and if you are by then are not dressed, you will freeze and be cold, so before that happen you want the wool to be on your body.

If you have been HERE and not started your inner dialogue, and NOT started talking with your friend how brave you were and who to tell and so on . . . .

You will now be filled with HAPPYNESS. Pure love. Nature is pressing on you.

So prepare to be loved, to feel love, to feel a warmth flow through you that nothing and no-one has given you before. So this is the WHY!

To feel being loved. And it can be repeated every day if you want (but the more often you do the longer you have to stay, but we are talking 7 minutes instead of 3 minutes, ha ha). The other benefits are also worthy additions.

LOVE

4. GOING IN THE FIRST TIME

METAPHORICALLY ONE CAN describe life as an ocean and you can live in (master) the sea in three ways.

1. You drown.
2. You swim
3. You walk on the water.

Here you are, mastering your fear and going to be really cold, painfully so for the first time.

On the place of your choosing, with a trusted friend at the waterfront you are ready. It may be that you did not find a friend to accompany you into the water, still if you get a trusted friend sitting quietly ashore it is OK. This is about YOU, this is not a shared experience anyway.

Anyway the water beckon to you. Your mind is set, you know you can do it. So take a minute, sit down and go through in your mind what you shall do; Undress, put the clothes so they are easy to put on again, walk down to water, enter water and walk into the water until you reach the chest level. If you are in a river or very shallow water, you have to walk to knee level and then lay down, never mind how, you need to be immersed in water to neck.

When you are ready, try to be still in mind, not follow your fantasies and thoughts, let nature absorb you.

So just do it, one step at a time, remember to breath deep and slow, take your time. Do things slowly, measured and be present in what you do. Do not let the pain swallow you, feel safe, feel prepared, you can do it. Try not to follow your thoughts, use mind to experience the body, the pain, the fear, the you.

You dip yourself and for each time it is easier, because you know you can do it. The pain will never leave you, even when in future you continue to do it, but the fear will leave you. The pain is necessary for making the body release the endorphins and the love, but even the pain after some times doing it – is not really present.

Coming out of the water you feel reborn, you know you will do it again and you feel full.

If you have read my book "A Handbook for Mastering Your (Inner) Life" you have a greater understanding of the mind and how to be still, but if you have not read it, the book is about how to stop the inner dialogue.

Here are some excerpts about what is a mind?

> Simply put, the mind is a "screen" that allows all your thinking / talking to yourself or imagination to be viewed, to be seen by your real "I" the soul. Most often we identify ourselves with the thoughts we have, but by training / mastering you can experience to mentally take "a step back" and "look" at your thoughts, so one sees the mind process.

> To use a symbol, the moon and the sun. If the sun is a symbol of God that gives light to the world and the moon reflects this light. This is the symbol of mastery, the mind becomes quiet and the light of God / rays of creativity / wisdom / reflect on our mind.

Why do I speak of the mind? Well it is because what you have experienced is all bout mind, about conquering fear and being present and still. Do read this chapter before doing it, specially if you are alone going into the water.

5. THIS IS IT

THE FINAL SAY on swimming in cold water is this; You can if you do it.

The chapters before is written to prepare you for wading into the icy waters, to tell you what you need to know since you don't have anybody with you that are experienced. It is a simple thing, most anybody can do it, but caution should be taken.

By swimming in cold water it brings you closer to nature, it makes you become an environmentalist and a carer of beaches. I always bring a bag and bring home garbage blown into the beach, in my opinion picking garbage is the truest prayer to the Creator that is known.

I wrote earlier that one can see the air at night

This is a thing to do for us that have time and place to go. You need a place in nature where there is dark, not light from the city and street-lights. You sit down and see into the forest or trees (I find this easiest), like seeing into a wall of green. Then you try to un-focuse your eyes, that is you try to focus between you and the trees. Think about those pictures that is created of dots and if you focus rightly you see a 3D figure. This is the same thing, the air is full of dark spots (it somehow remind me of "Dust" in the "Golden Compass" trilogy by Phillip Pullman or what is called dark matter.

You may ask what is the point, well I may ask what will it lead to? Maybe it is possible to step up unto the air, I don't know, maybe you are the one doing it.

I am of the opinion that there is actually a right behavior in all situations, but it is not predetermined, it is acknowledged as the action takes place. To reach such a living realization the mind should be trained and it can be trained.

6. THE SECRET OF THE VALØ STONES (THE SECRET STONES OF THE VIKINGS)

What is a valø stone?

NORWAY IS A very old country and has been covered in deep ice in the past. There have been times that the thickness of the ice have been up to 3-4 km thick. Today there are more than 1500 glaciers in Norway. These huge layers of ice grind down the mountains beneath them, breaking loose huge boulders and slowly grinding them down and some turns into the valø stones after millions of years. So from a big rock it is ground down to about the size of your fist or smaller (they vary greatly in size and colour).

They may seem like any round rock (we call them dinosaur eggs), but they are all different and all have different properties due to size, inner structure and form. One can say that they are "alive" in a certain sense. But two very different valø stones in appearance can have the same properties for that which we will use them for.

So not all stones are a valø stones, and not all are "alive". So finding the live ones is an art and skill, and not a easy task to do.

How does a valø stone work?

As some of you may know there is an energy centre in the belly, you may know this from experience of fear and anxiety; it is felt in the stomach. One may say that many emotions live in the stomach and upset your calmness and well-being.

There is a "centre" or "opening" located three finger widths down from the bellybutton, and by following the simple instructions and by placing a valø stone on this "opening" for half an hour, the valø stone will "slow" you down and can lead you towards inner health. It is like taking a short journey daily, to achieve this inner health.

The energy of a valø stone.

This is a holistic approach to well-being. Stored in a valø stone is four kinds of energy; Mechanical-, Chemical-, Radiant and Nuclear energy. It may sound new to you that a stone can have energy stored inside, and it is not easily proven.

- The Mechanical energy is the force that moves objects. In the case of the valø stone the great forces that have created them are stored as a potential inside.
- The Chemical energy is when the valø stone is moved on your skin.
- Radiant energy is the force that created the stone in the beginning from the lava and it molten origin. This vital energy (like the one from the sun) is still present as a shadow of its past.
- Nuclear energy is the force of atoms and its smaller particles. All things created vibrate and to an extent moves, so does the force of the valø stone.

The healing power of a valø stone.

A valø stone will help you achieve inner health, with translates to outer radiance. The women will like this aspect a lot, as it makes them more radiant and attractive. Also it charges them with greater harmony and purpose.

For men it takes the edge of their unease and build power. Since they slowly stop loosing vital energy, this translates into stronger sexual drive and mental purpose.

Since the stones harmonize your energy, it can slow and stop the drain, so the healing of your energy body can commence. Some of its curative power can help and cure many disorders related to energy loss like; Poor blood circulation, nervousness, mental instability, negative thought patterns, lack of sexual vitality and many more.

Do *believe* in what you DO, take faith serious, believe in yourself and have empathy. Your body is not a machine, it is the outer layer for your soul to experience the world. There are many layers and the energy body is the form that hold your physical body together. Strengthening the energy body with the valø stone gives untold benefits, so give yourself this precious gift and may it give you the most needed boost in your life.

History.

The valø stones have been used in secret for more than 3000 years, the Vikings chieftains and their wives used them more than a 1000 years ago. It is not a known fact as they never shared an edge or a personal power.

Today most people in Norway believe only in aspirin and antibiotics. What a shame.

How is it identified?

Finding the valø stones have been a secret inside a few families and past on to the eldest son in each generation. By a certain method I choose a stone to an individual.

I have in late years identified five major stone-types, or resonant group of stones. I can find the stones and identify which group it belong to, but how to match them to the correct person from a distance?

I knew plants also have a resonance and the plant-kingdom is between man and mineral. This led me to research into how plants could help identifying the five major groups of people. My research led me to Dr. Sharifah Hafizah (Ph.D) and her research into aromatherapy. She developed five mixtures where the five major personalities resonance. So with her method one can identify what person or resonance one belong to, and I have pre-matched and marked the stones and as such you can be sure of getting the full benefit of a correct valø stone matched to you.

There are two ways to use the valø stone – Floating and Energy. They are both fully described and are really easy to do, and the benefits are great.

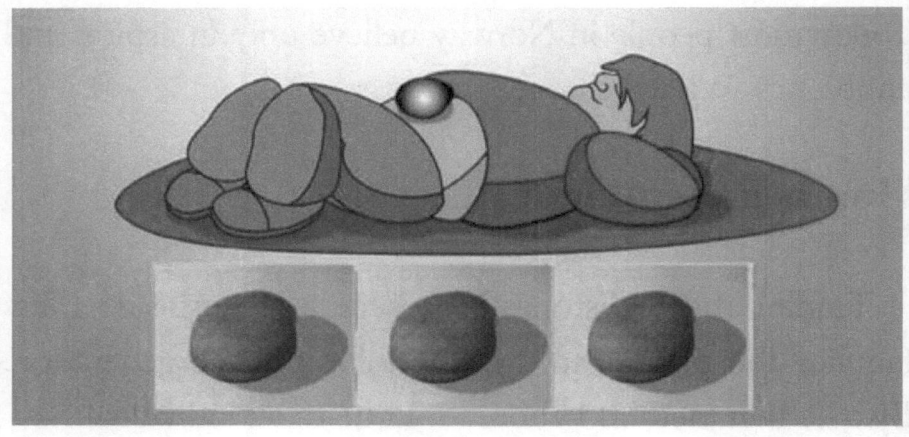

Preparation for use.

As you may know there is an energy centre in the belly, you may know this from experience of fear and anxiety; it is felt in the stomach. One may say that many emotions live in the stomach and upset your calmness, well-being and drain your energy.

This "centre" or "opening" is located three finger widths down from the bellybutton is where you place your valø stone for half an hour.

You start with placing your valø stone in a container with warm or hot water. Put the palm of your right hand where the "energy opening is and gently move it in a circle counterclockwise for a minute. The circle the size of your valø stone. You can use a few drops of cold pressed virgin olive oil and the exchange will be softer then.

Lay down on your back on a bed or in a recliner, make it very comfortable. Then place the valø stone gently on the centre of the energy opening. If the valø stone is too hot wait until it is warm but comfortable (it should not burn you or give blisters, only be so warm that its presence is clearly felt).

Take a few deep breaths, deep abdominal breathing (when you breath in your stomach moves out and when you breath out your stomach moves in). If it is cold or the stone rolls off, put a towel or cloth to keep your valø stone in place. Make sure you can still breath deeply and unrestricted.

Then you have to decide if you want to do either of the two exercises; Floating or Energy. Also start you first time with only five to ten minutes, extend your length of time slowly until you do the full 30 minutes. Make sure you have someone to wake you up the first times you use the valø stone as its power is strong, and you can experience a disturbed sleep with it on you. But do not fear, it just start making you healthy, vibrant and strong.

Remember strength is not given, it is claimed. When energy is retained, the energy body expand and get stronger.

Floating exercise.

The floating exercise slows down the nervous energy and make you start to relax fully. This is why it is so easy to fall asleep in the beginning. Falling asleep can make you have unpleasant dreams, but do not fear. Read the paragraph called conquering dreams and learn it by heart. In the first few times it is better to do the exercise in the presence of a friend, so he or she can gently wake you up if you fall asleep. Later on you will welcome the sleep during the exercise, but then it will seldom come.

So sit or lay down comfortably, put your right palm-center 3 finger widths below the belly button, this is the energy opening (some call it the Hule). Place the valø stone with the centre of the stone on the energy opening. If it the valø stone roll off when you breath, put a cloth or towel around waist, but make sure the valø stone is in place and in contact with your skin.

Then you are all set and ready to go (metaphysically speaking).

You close your eyes and "imagine" that you breath through through your valø stone, through your energy opening (the Hule). You "imagine" that the "air" flows in through the valø stone, though the Hule, like a wave going through your body to the top of your head and then reside down and out of your body through the Hule.

Think of the wave flowing in and out. Breath slow and gently, deep abdominal breathing, your stomach move out when breathing in and your stomach move in when your breathing breathing out.

As easy as that, but yes following you "breath" in and out of your body is not so easy in the beginning. You forget yourself, you get out of breath because you formulate what you do and by the time you have the "breath" get to your head you need to take another breath.

DO NOT WORRY!

This exercise is easy to understand, and for most of us difficult to do in the beginning. Look at any person that is good in anything, either an athlete or a musician, they all train daily for years. So it is for us, doing this exercise daily will slowly improve our skill and even with small daily effort we will have small gains that is visible for us and our surroundings.

So keep at it and the rewards and changes will soon be felt do to your continuous effort.

Remember your goals; to be more energetic, to be a more vital and whole person, be calm, have more sexual energy and be a more vibrant and attractive person.

Lofty goals all of them, and they can be yours with daily effort.

Energy exercise.

The energy exercise boost your energy and make you energy body expand.

I assume you have read the paragraph "Preparation for use", and in any case do reread it to fully understand it.

Reread also the paragraph "Conquering dreams" and learn it by heart. In the first few times it is better to do even this exercise in the presence of a friend, so he or she can gently wake you up if you fall asleep.

So sit down comfortably in a chair or a recliner, put on the oil and rub counterclockwise on the centre which is located 3 finger widths below the belly button. Then you put the flat of your right hand palm over the Hule on your bare skin. Gently move your hand in a small circle with your palm on your skin counterclockwise 99 times. This energize the hand. Then you hold your hand as a cup and hold your balls (a woman put the palm flat on the skin of the vagina) for 1-3 minutes, this make the energy flow into the sexual organ.

Then you put your valø stone on the Hule. If it the valø stone roll off when you breath, put a cloth or towel around waist, but make sure the valø stone is in place and in contact with your skin.

You put your hands together in as if you would clap your hands, palm to palm and fingers to fingers. Find a comfortable position for your arms and then for 30 minutes you clap your hands while you do the internal "breathing" like the Floating exercise.

So you close your eyes and "imagine" that you breath through through your valø stone, through your energy opening (the Hule). You "imagine" that the "air" flows in through the valø stone, though the Hule, like a wave going through your body to the top of your head and then reside down and out of your body through the Hule, and at the same time you clap your hands.

This is not so easy, and your arms may tire in the beginning, so start with 5 minutes and every day increase with one minute until you can do the full 30 minutes.

When your time is up, lift your arms gently straight up, palms facing forward and feel the energy flowing down from your hands and arms into your body.

The moment you lift up your arms is VERY important, do not waste your precious generated energy. So be fully aware of the sensations of the energy flowing into your body.

Later when you become more able to be aware and concentrated, you can direct this energy to any place in your body that is weak, sick or need special attention and healing.

Remember your goals; to be more energetic, to be a more vital and whole person, be calm, have more sexual energy and be a more vibrant and attractive person.

Lofty goals all of them, and they can be yours with daily effort.

Conquering dreams.

Dreams are just that, dreams. Yes there are dreams of value, dreams sent to you for knowledge and guidance, but most dreams are just like a release of anxiety or hopes. So to get rid of the useless dreams, those that scare or confuse you, you need to do a conscious action in your dream. This conscious action can be anything, but the easiest is to lift and look at the palms of your hands.

Do it now, lift up and look at the palms of your hands, really take a good look. This action is what you will need to do inside your dream. So try to wake up inside your dream, to wake up is to do an conscious action inside your dream – then you control them.

Most people stop dreaming after doing their first conscious action in their dreams. Do not worry, those dreams are just figment of imagination and of no value, dreams of value will come when they come, be patient if you want them.

More energy can make that a possibility. Some will have no dreams and at any rate dreams fade, only presence remain.

Belief in doing.

Do *believe* in what you DO, take faith serious, believe in yourself and have empathy. Your body is not a machine, it is the outer layer for your soul to experience the world. There are many layers and the energy body is the form that hold your physical body together. Strengthening the energy body with the valø stone gives untold benefits, so give yourself this precious gift and may it give you the most needed boost in your life.

Disclaimer.

Without the valø stone as they have the needed balancing effect the effect is less, but you can try to find a stone on the beach that you feel connected to and take it from there.

If you order a stone from me there will be no refund, as the valø stone is picked and set to YOU. We would need to communicate to identify what person you are to fit the correct stone to you. See inside for email.

If you for some reason will not use your valø stone it can not be returned. But it will lay patiently waiting for you to commence that healing process.

I have never heard any negative experiences from using the valø stone, but people can blame any experiences on them, so it is prudent I say you do it on your own risk and all exercises should not be started without consulting your physician.

. . . .

My research led me to Dr. Sharifah "Ezza" Hafizah (Ph.D) and her research into aromatherapy. She developed the five mixtures where the five major personalities resonance. So with her method one can identify what person or resonance one belong to. You can easily identify what person you belong to and then I can here identify the stone for that particular resonance. I match and mark the stones and as such you can be sure of getting the full benefit of a correct Valo stone matched to you.

So many thanks to Ezza for helping me with that, because if not for her method I needed to physically hold the person and the stone to feel the match.

7. EPILOGUE

AFTER DOING THE cold water rejuvenation and the valø stones for a while you may feel new in a sense, reborn even, open to the flow of experience from our mythical past has reached you in this present.

I wish for you a life where you have an eternal interest and curiosity, optimism and belief in that you can search and find answers. All the answers you may find are not "the final answer" to any question, but answers that lead to new ways of "seeing" things and to ever new questions.

You may start to reflect on these, and find arguments in favor of:

1. A Creator
2. Acting friendly and inclusive
3. Take care of the environment and nature
4. Why quality is important

You do this to have insights, to have mindfulness.

From Norway, the land of fjords, glaziers and valø stones, I wish you a blessed, healthy and prosperous life.

Warm regards from mr. Borge Bahr Naseer Blatind

WHY WOULD ANYBODY IN THEIR RIGHT MIND GO INTO REALLY COLD WATER YOU MAY ASK?

THE PAIN AND fear you experience going into cold water is immense the first time you do it. So most people would only dip their toe or finger in the water and run for warm clothing.

So why would anybody in their right mind go into the cold water?

The short explanation is you will look and feel younger and more vibrant. There are many other hidden benefits and rejuvenation that you will experience if you do it the right way.

This short book tell you how to do it, and what to experience. I will also tell you about an old Norwegian healing method that you can do at home to make you even more vibrant.

YOU CAN IF YOU DO IT!

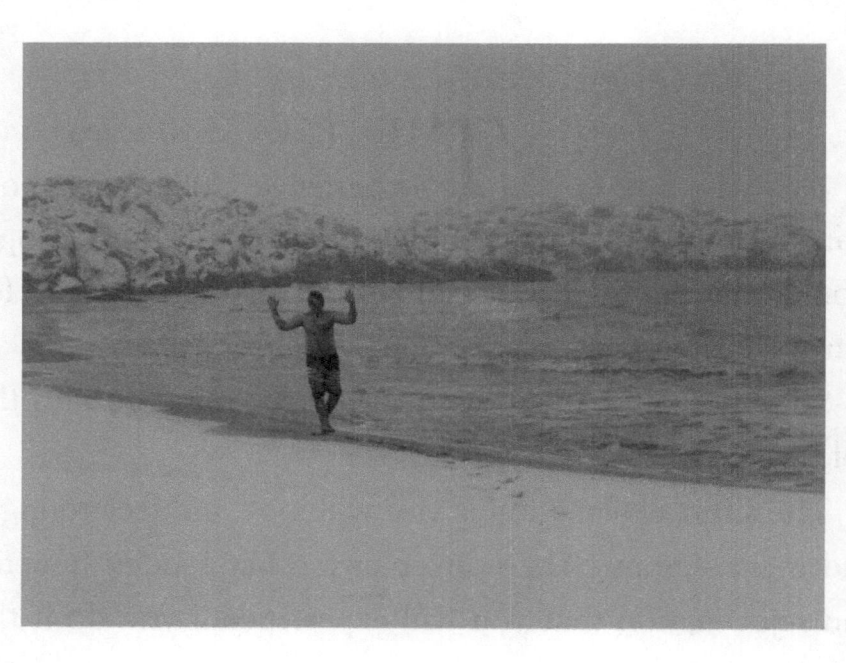

www.ingramcontent.com/pod-product-compliance
Lightning Source LLC
Chambersburg PA
CBHW030540290526
45786CB00004B/1799